SIR JOHN WILL[illegible]

Bart., M.[illegible]

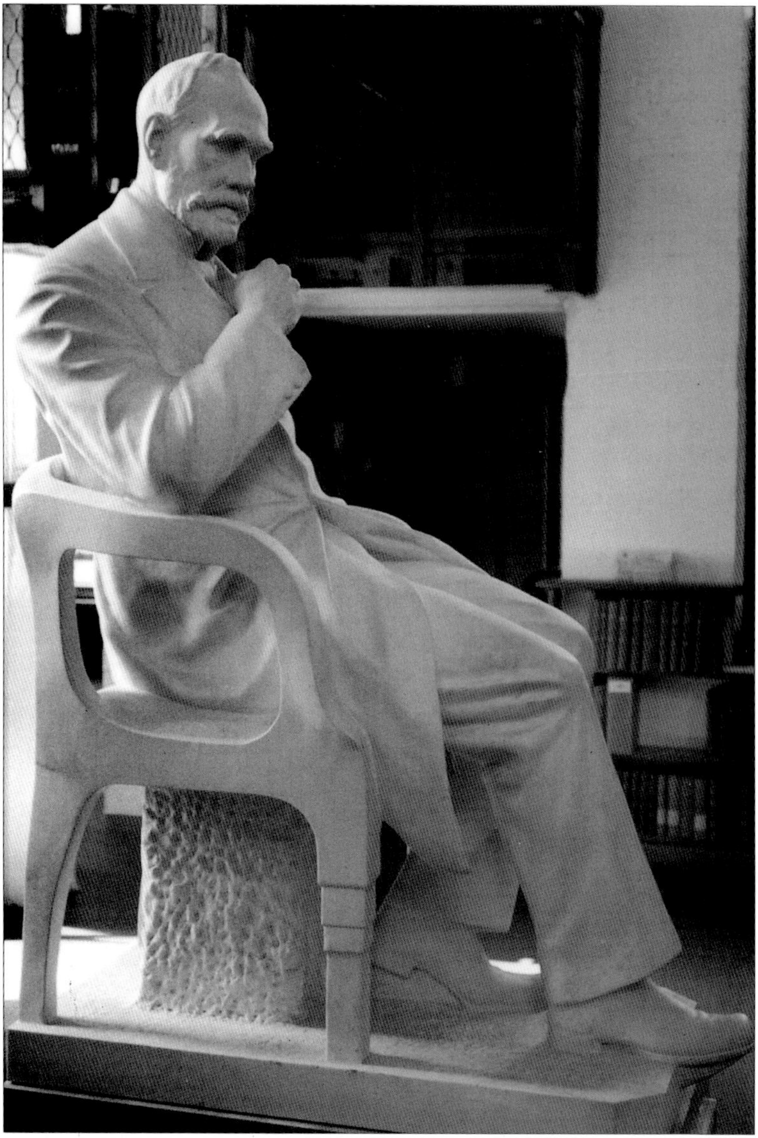

Sir John Williams, Bart., the marble sculpture by Mario Rutelli.

SIR JOHN WILLIAMS

Bart., M.D.

1840-1926

Founder-President
of the
National Library of Wales

'A singularly great man'

Robert Brinley Jones

The Drovers Press
2007

Published in 2007 by
The Drovers Press
Drovers Farm, Porthyrhyd, Llanwrda
Carmarthenshire, SA19 8DF

ISBN 978-0-9557541-0-4

A CIP catalogue record for this book is available from the British Library.

Printed and bound in Wales by
Dinefwr Press Ltd.
Rawlings Road, Llandybie
Carmarthenshire, SA18 3YD

To my wife

STEPHANIE

". . . mewn gwerthfawrogiad"

Contents

Preface

In November 1996 I was elected President of the National Library of Wales. I had known the institution years earlier as a research student and later as a member of its Council. In November 2007 I retire after an extraordinary period of pleasure and privilege of serving this great cultural institution. I shall never forget my indebtedness to the support of staff, of Council and Board members during my period of office: I record my gratitude to them all. Diolch o waelod calon.

From the start I was aware of the enormous contribution made by the first President, Sir John Williams and in this year of 2007 when we celebrate the centenary of the granting of the Charter to the Library it seemed appropriate to re-tell, briefly, the story of his life and the extent of his contribution.

In preparing this essay I have been fortunate in having ready assistance from my colleagues in the Library: the Librarian, Andrew Green, has been particularly helpful and I thank him, too, for his permission to use illustrations from the Library's collections. I acknowledge, with gratitude, valuable comments from Dr T. G. Davies, Professor J. D. R. Thomas and Professor N. McIntyre on particular aspects of the work. I thank Mrs Margaret Davies for preparing my script for publication and the printers for their cooperation.

October 2007 *R B.J.*

I

Beginnings

Sir John Williams, baronet, obstetrician, court physician, principal founder and most generous benefactor of the National Library of Wales, was born on 6 November 1840, at his maternal grandparents' home, Beili, Gwynfe, Llangadog, Carmarthenshire where his mother had returned for her confinement. Mother and child went back to the nearby family semi-upland tenant-holding, Blaenllynant, when John was a few weeks old. His parents had married in 1833 and John was the third son and fourth of five children. His father was David Williams (1802-1842), farmer and Congregationalist minister at nearby Bethlehem, Llangadog, who also had charge of the cause at Carmel, Llansadwrn; he had been ordained in 1838. David Williams died of typhoid fever, leaving three children, a daughter having died in infancy; there was one son yet to be born. John's mother was Eleanor (1807-1895), eldest of twelve children. Her father, David Jones of Beili, Gwynfe, was a farmer and freeholder, a powerful personality with a strong belief in the value of education. In consequence, Eleanor was sent for lessons to John Davies of Glanclydach, held in a schoolroom in Gwynfe. Later she went to another school near Glantywi in the Bethlehem, Llangadog area and, then, at the age of twelve attended a girls' school at Merthyr Tydfil,

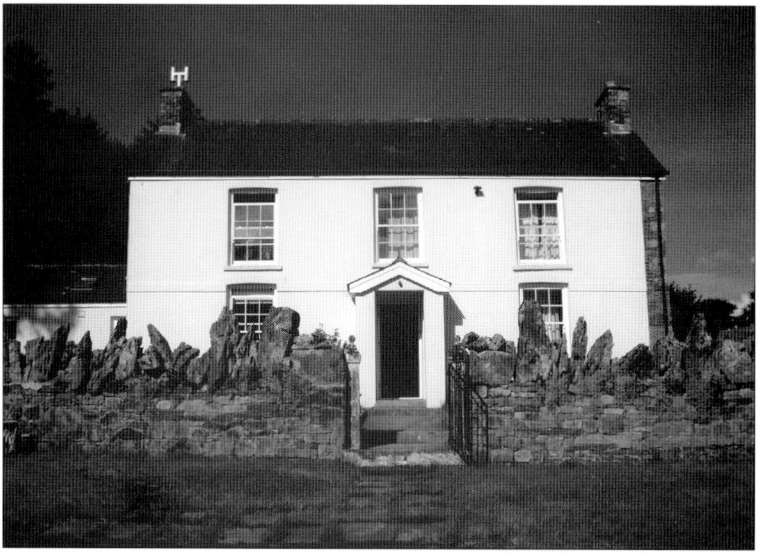

Blaenllynant (as it is today).
(Photographs by Donald Jones).

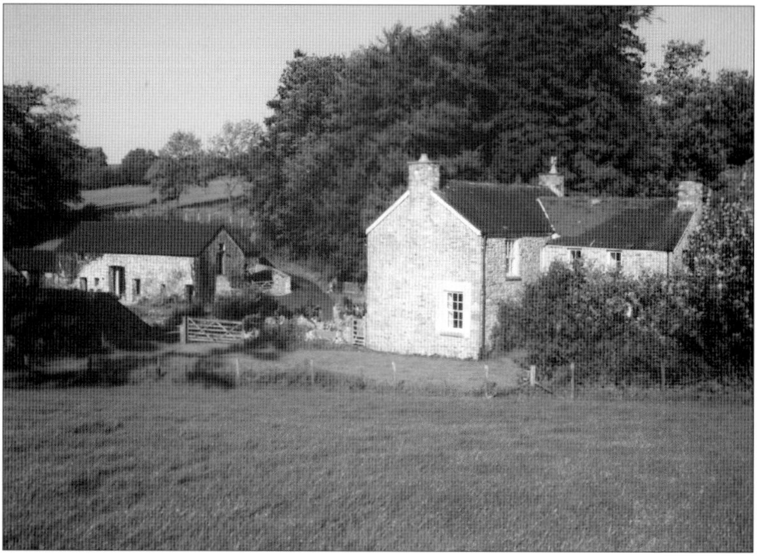

residing with her mother's sister there. It was a superior education for girls of her day and background and it was to inform the upbringing of her sons.

After her husband's death Eleanor continued with the help of family and servants, to work the farm at Blaenllynant: she instilled in her household strict religious obser-

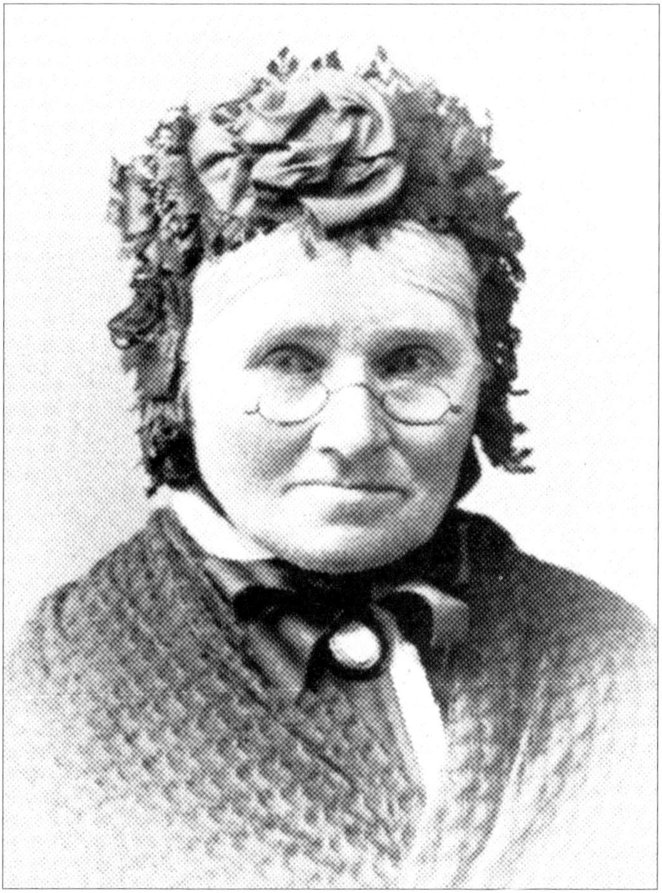

Eleanor Williams (in later life).

vance and a respect for education. She was a keen reader and taught her servants to read and write Welsh and English: significantly, among the household listed in the Census of 1841, including four servants, was 'William Morris, 18, Schoolmaster'. She was to remain a strong influence on John Williams for the whole of his life: he referred to her as his 'guide'. In 1885 he established a scholarship entitled 'The Eleanor Williams Exhibition', enabling local boys to continue their education at a Higher-grade school 'such as the Welsh Collegiate Institution, Llandovery, or Christ's College, Brecon'. Nathaniel, the son born after his father's death, was to compose a tribute to their mother – '*Byr-gofiant am Mrs Eleanor Williams, Talardd, Llandilo (Blaenllynant gynt)*': it was published in 1898. Eleanor died on 30 March, 1895.

II

Early Education

As a child, John attended lessons locally and at Sunday school and then proceeded to a dissenting day-school held in the schoolroom of Bethlehem Chapel some three miles away from his home. The school was conducted by the

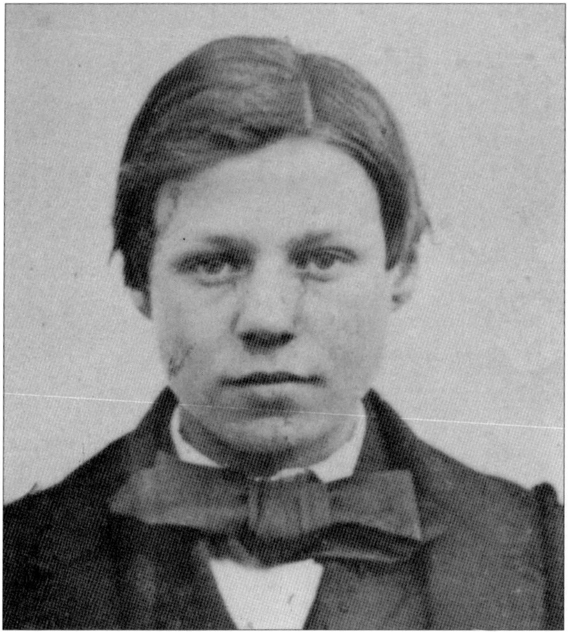

Young John Williams.

Reverend D. Davies and was supported by payments from parents and subscriptions from local farmers. John's family were staunch members of the Congregationalist cause – Jerusalem at the start and when Capel Maen, the daughter-church was opened in 1853, they joined it. John's brothers, David and Nathaniel both became chapel secretaries and John was later to preach there. He remembered his childhood years on the banks of Afon Meilwch, a tributary of the River Tywi with much pleasure and claimed that they had prepared him well for his future life – 'the effects have been my mainstay during the rest of my career', he recalled in 1900.

In 1855 John left for the Normal School at Swansea with the intention of preparing for the Nonconformist ministry. The Church Book of Capel Maen records that his membership there was transferred to Ebenezer, Swansea, in that year. The school had previously been home to a training college for teachers, inspired by the Nonconformist 'Voluntary' school movement. It had been sited at Brecon originally, with Evan Davies (1826-1872), born at Gelli-tyddyndu in the parish of Llanycrwys, Carmarthenshire, as head; it then moved to Swansea but when it faltered as a result of the collapse of the Voluntaryist movement and financial difficulties Evan Davies continued to run it as a private venture school. Evan Davies was to be John's mentor: he himself had been educated at the Froodvale Academy, a well-regarded preparatory school in Pumsaint, near Llandovery. He had made a marked impression there; the head, The Reverend Dr William Davies, listed him as one of the 'preachers who were under my tuition' and one of his contemporaries was to comment: 'It was generally regarded that Mr Evan Davies was king of the school for ever . . .

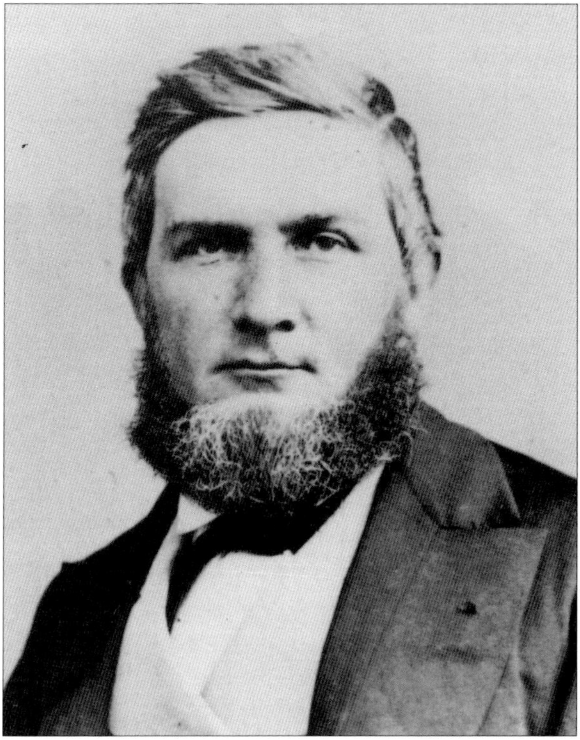

Dr Evan Davies.

There was no mention of anyone like him from the start, and no sensible one expected anyone like him to appear again' (tr). Evan Davies left there for Bristol and then the University of Glasgow with the intention of entering the Nonconformist ministry. (He was to receive the LL.D. degree from Glasgow in 1858.) Evan Davies had recognised very special gifts in John Williams but, rather than pursuing a course leading to ordination, was to encourage him to pursue a scientific career. With that in mind, John proceeded to the University of Glasgow in 1857.

III

Glasgow

The University of Glasgow was founded in 1451: it was set 'where the air is mild, victuals are plentiful, and a great store of other things pertaining to the use of man is found'. It suffered troubled years from time to time but, with the American tobacco trade in the eighteenth century and the cotton trade in the nineteenth century, the city gained prosperity. Certainly with the prohibitions experienced by dissenters, the university was to attract promising students from Scotland, England, Ireland and Wales. Welshmen found it an agreeable place.

David Daniel Davis (1777-1841), from the parish of Llandyfaelog, Carmarthen, had proceeded via the Dissenting Academy of Northampton to the University of Glasgow. His original intention – like that of John Williams – was to train for the Nonconformist ministry, but his sights turned to Medicine. He was to become the first Professor of Midwifery at the University of London in 1827. He was the Physician Accoucheur attending the Duchess of Kent at the birth of Queen Victoria in 1819. He was to favour more active intervention in childbirth and encouraged the use of forceps in obstetrics and improved the design of instruments to assist childbirth: he constructed five different patterns of forceps. He was a prolific writer on matters of obstetrics: his *Elements of Operative Midwifery*, 1825 and *The Principles and Practice of Obstetric Medicine* . . . 1836 crystallised his theories, teaching and research.

(Sir) William Milbourne James (1807-1881), born in Merthyr Tydfil was educated at Glasgow and then Lincoln's Inn: he was appointed Lord Justice of Appeal in 1870.

William Morgan (1818-1884) of Henllan Amgoed, Carmarthenshire went from Froodvale Academy to Hackney College, London and then to Glasgow: he was to gain considerable prominence in the fields of education, equality and religious and political freedom.

One of John Williams' near contemporaries, (Sir) Henry Jones (1852-1922) from Llangernyw, Denbighshire, was to enter Glasgow in 1875 and later, in 1894, was appointed Professor of Philosophy there, succeeding Edward Caird who had been an inspiration to Owen Morgan Edwards during his sojourn at Glasgow 1883-1884. Edward Caird's brother, John (later to become Principal) was minister of Park Church. His sermons together with those of another distinguished divine, Alexander Raleigh impressed young John Williams during his time there.

John Williams was to remain at Glasgow for one agreeable and successful year, studying Mathematics under Professor Hugh Blackburn. But Swansea beckoned again – maybe because of financial pressure, maybe because he needed to be nèarer home, maybe because the possibility of testing another discipline suggested itself to him. In July 1859 he was apprenticed to W. H. Michael, surgeon and apothecary and Dr Ebenezer Davies. His apprenticeship indenture bound him for five years to learn the art and science of Medicine and Surgery . . . but he was to stay for two years only.

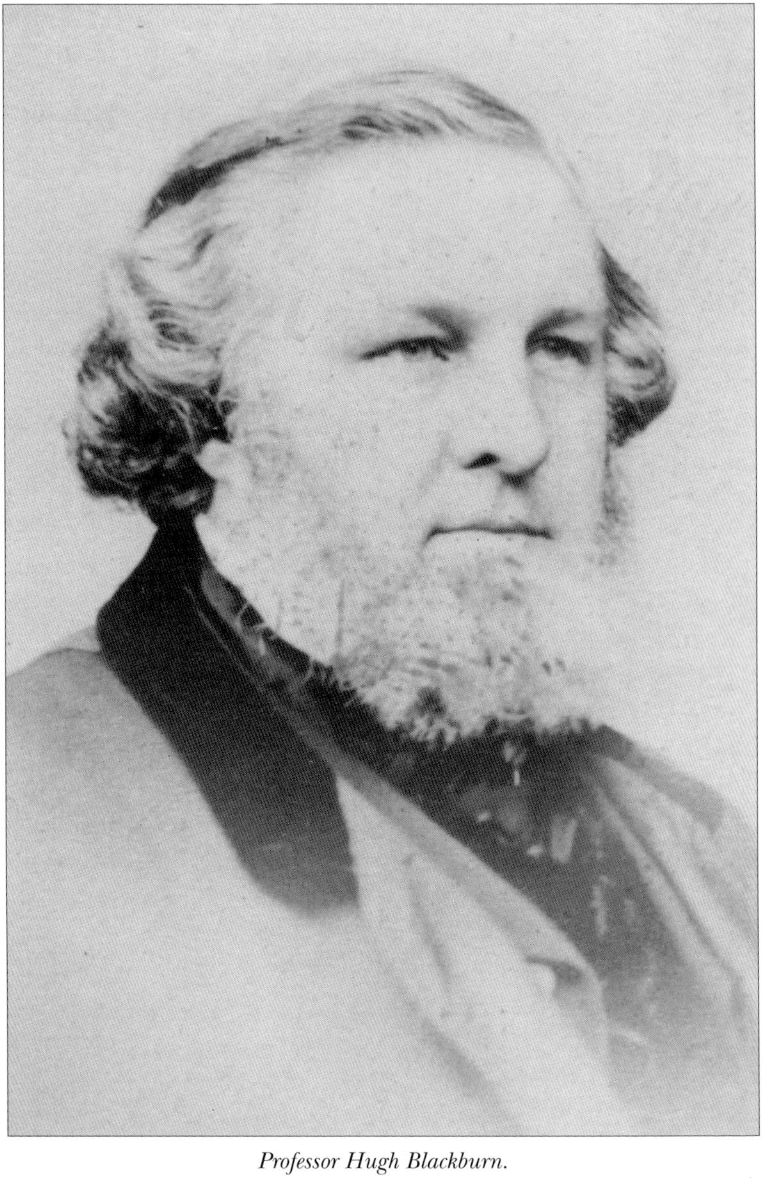

Professor Hugh Blackburn.

IV

University College Hospital, London

John Williams had found his niche. Glasgow, whose university he knew and whose well-respected private medical college, Anderson College, dating from the first quarter of the nineteenth century was gaining a reputation, might have enticed him back there but London was to be his choice. In his twenty-first year, John Williams entered University College Hospital: it was a hospital that attracted other Welshmen who distinguished themselves, among them C. J. Blasius Williams (1805-1889) who is reputed to have given the first complete description of mitral stenosis, Timothy Richards Lewis (1841-1886), a leading figure in tropical pathology (whose manuscripts are in the National Library), Ernest Jones (1879-1958), the psychoanalyst, (Sir) Thomas Lewis (1881-1945), cardiologist and Hugh Morriston Davies (1879-1965) a pioneer in thoracic surgery.

John was to study under William Jenner, who had been Professor of Pathological Anatomy there since 1849 and physician to the hospital: he was Holme Professor of Clinical Medicine at the college when John entered and in 1863 was appointed Professor of Principles and Practice of Medicine. He was one of those who established the distinct identities of typhus and typhoid fever and had attended Prince Albert before he died of the fever in 1861, the year in which

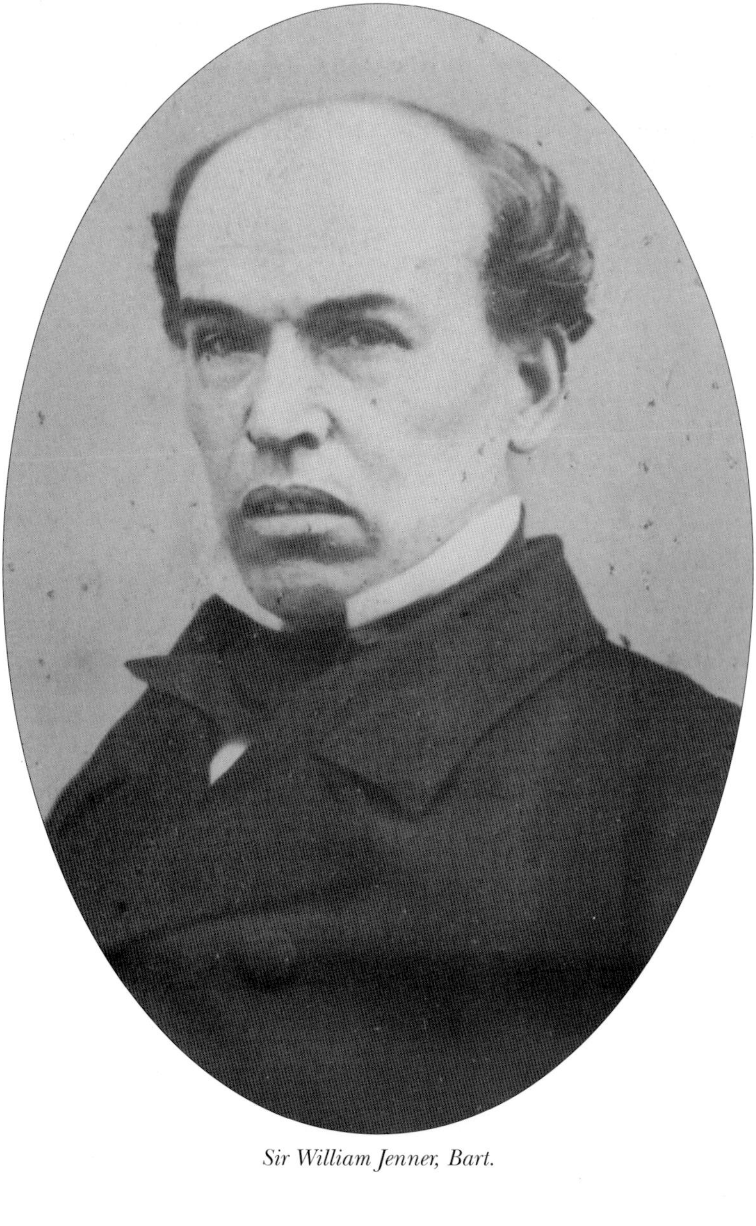

Sir William Jenner, Bart.

John had entered University College Hospital. Jenner's expertise was close to John's heart since his father had died, young, from typhoid fever. Jenner was regarded as being the outstanding consultant of his time and an unforgettable clinical teacher. The notebook still exists in John Williams' hand of lectures delivered by Jenner in 1863/4: he was to be a formidable influence on John Williams.

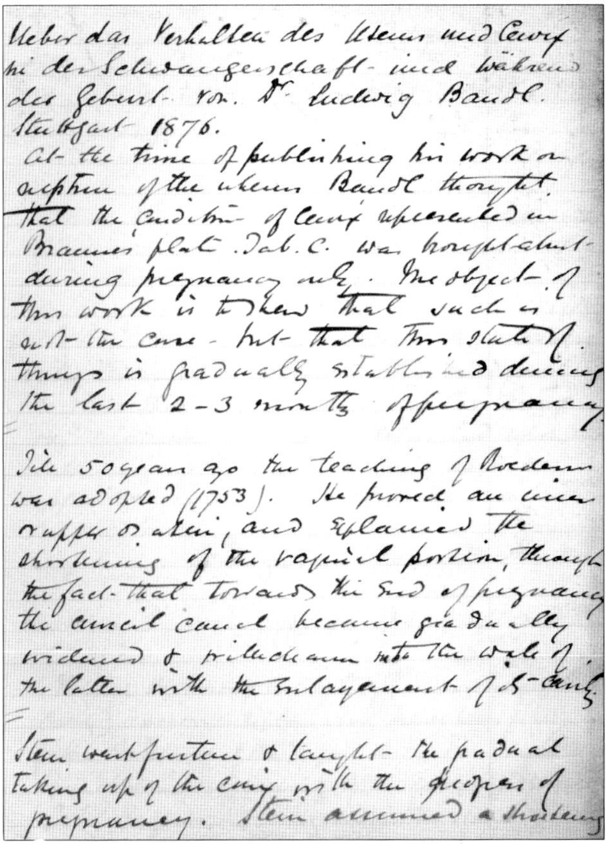
Ueber das Verhalten des Uterus und Cervix bei der Schwangerschaft und während der Geburt. von Dr Ludwig Bandl. Stuttgart 1876.
At the time of publishing his work on rupture of the uterus Bandl thought that the condition of cervix represented in Braune's plate Tab. C. was brought about during pregnancy only. The object of this work is to shew that such is not the case - but that this state of things is gradually established during the last 2-3 months of pregnancy.

Till 50 years ago the teaching of Roederer was adopted (1753). He proved an inner or upper os uteri, and explained the shortening of the vaginal portion, through the fact that towards the end of pregnancy the cervical canal became gradually widened & pulled up into the walls of the latter with the enlargement of its cavity.

Stein went further & taught the gradual taking up of the cervix with the progress of pregnancy. Stein assumed a shortening

Notes in John Williams' hand.

Another of his tutors was Sydney Ringer, only five years his senior: he was to compile *A Handbook of Therapeutics* in 1869 (a volume which ran to its thirteenth edition in 1897). Ringer was to be Holme Professor of Clinical Medicine 1887-1900. (In the same year, 1887, John Williams would be elected Professor of Obstetric Medicine.)

John Williams completed his medical studies having won the Silver Medal for Chemistry, 1861-1862 and for Anatomy and Physiology, 1862-1863, taking the Gold Medal for Pathological Anatomy, 1864-1865. He gained the degree of Doctor of Medicine of the University of London in December 1867: he was licensed to practise Medicine.

Having held resident posts at the Brompton Chest Hospital and the Great Ormond Street Hospital for Sick Children, he returned to Swansea, to 13 Cradock Street, as a general practitioner after a very distinguished student career and considerable and varied hospital training and experience.

V

Medical Posts

London, however, was enticing and in February 1872 John Williams was appointed Assistant Obstetric Physician at University College Hospital. (It was the year in which the university college opened in Aberystwyth.) In April of the same year at Libanus Chapel, Morriston, he married Mary Elizabeth Anne Hughes, 'Lizzie' whose bardic name was

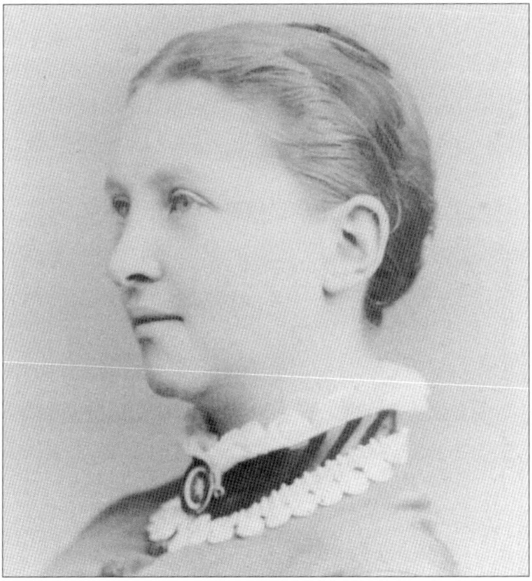

'Lizzie'.

Morvudd Glantawe. She was nine years his junior, the only child of Richard Hughes JP of Ynystawe, near Swansea, successful and respected industrialist, partner in the Landore Tinplate Works. Lizzie's uncle was the Reverend Michael D. Jones of Bala, ardent nationalist and one of the prime-movers in establishing the Welsh Colony in Patagonia. (A piece of the gold medal which John had won for Pathology was punched and used for his bride's wedding-ring.) They moved to London, to 28 Harley Street. John gained the M.R.C.P. (London) in the following year and in 1879 he was elected F.R.C.P. (Providing a break from his arduous schedule of duties, he and his wife made a tour of the West Indies in 1881.)

John Williams was promoted Obstetric Physician in 1883, a position he held jointly with William Morse Graily Hewitt (1828-1893): he distinguished himself as a pioneer expert obstetrician and a reputable 'surgical' gynaecologist. In 1879 he had been joint secretary of the Obstetrical Society of London and wrote to the General Medical Council suggesting that a more detailed study of Obstetrics should become a compulsory part of the undergraduate medical course in Britain. For two years, 1887-1888, he was President of that society.

In the controversies among late Victorian obstetricians he was an ally of James Matthews Duncan (1826-1890), taking a middle view as between those practitioners who were averse to operation and those who favoured it. John was himself a skilled operator and his successor in the chair of Obstetric Medicine, Herbert Ritchie Spencer (1860-1941) regarded it as one of Williams' achievements that obstetricians secured the right to operate at the hospitals of other medical schools. Williams was also known as an

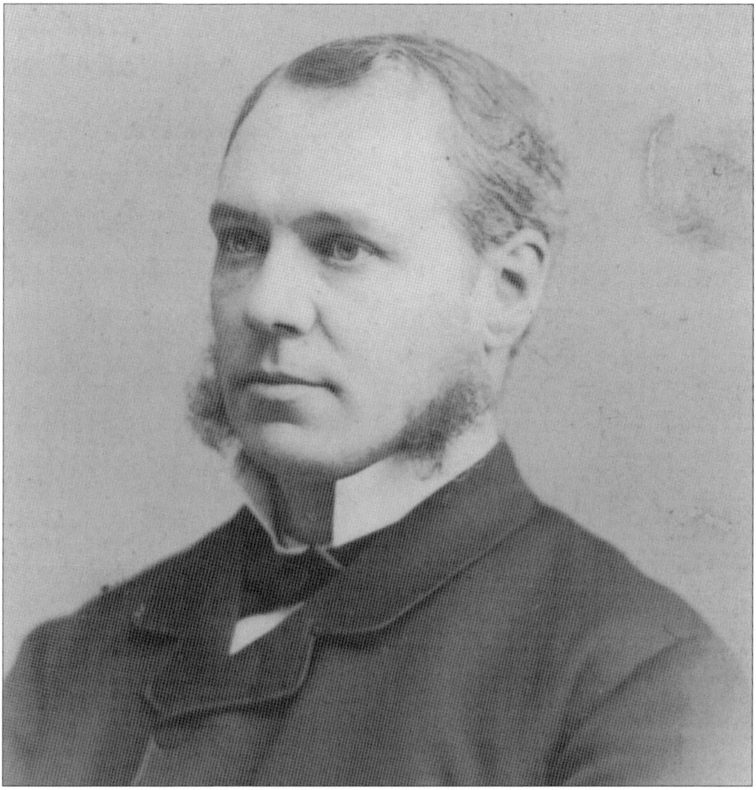

Dr John Williams.

enthusiastic disciple of Joseph Lister's antiseptic system in the prevention and treatment of infection. It was his friend, Marcus Beck (nephew of Lister), who had introduced the system into University College Hospital in 1869: Duncan and Williams were the apostles of Listerism in this respect. Spencer was to comment, 'It was due to his early employment of the antiseptic system that Williams largely owed his success in Obstetrics and Gynaecology'. (Occasionally John

Williams would attend medical meetings in Swansea and in 1880 at one such meeting he gave an address on 'Antiseptics in Midwifery'.) Iorwerth Hughes Jones was to sum up his significance in these words: 'The special contribution of Sir John Williams to the progress of medicine was his immediate application of Lister's discoveries on antiseptics to the practice of obstetrics, and then, as an operating gynaecologist to the surgery of the abdomen, made possible by these new methods. Further it was he who first combined in one person, the practice of obstetrics and the skill of an operating gynaecologist'.

It was said that his influence upon Obstetrics and Gynaecology arose even more from his personal character than from his scientific work. He gained a reputation as a popular clinical teacher who instilled the practice of careful note-taking. He was not a great public speaker but what he said was sensible, pertinent and direct. One of his distinguished pupils, Thomas Watts Eden described him as 'the greatest teacher of his time'. And John's assistant, Thomas Barlow, said of him, 'He was a sound teacher and a staunch friend to all his students, and he rapidly acquired a distinguished position in London amongst consultants'. His students were to hold key appointments in various hospitals at home and abroad.

Williams was a cautious, critical researcher and did not publish widely: like his teacher, William Jenner, his publications were few but were significant and of good judgement. His main contributions are to be found in the *Transactions of the Obstetrical Society*, his Harveian Lecture on 'Cancer of the Uterus' and in the Cavendish Lecture on 'Ovarian Tumours complicating Pregnancy'. He became the first chairman of the *Journal of Obstetrics and Gynaecology of the*

British Empire and was a member of the General Medical Council from 1901 to 1911 when he was involved in reforming the teaching of Gynaecology and Midwifery. He was active in the promotion of the education of midwives . . . but he demonstrated a wider interest, too. In October 1900 he delivered an 'Introductory Address on the training of body and mind for the profession of Medicine' given at the commencement of the Winter Session of the Faculty of Medicine of the University College of South Wales: it was published in the *British Medical Journal* on 13 October 1900. He was elected to many professional bodies both in the United Kingdom and abroad, including Berlin, Moscow and Boston, Massachusetts. In 1890 he delivered the opening address in Obstetrics at the International Medical Congress at Berlin on 'The total extirpation of the uterus by the vagina'. (This was later published in *The Lancet.*)

In 1887 he had succeeded Hewitt as Professor of Obstetric Medicine and in 1893 he was Consulting Obstetric Physician at University College Hospital. He served concurrently at the General Lying-in Hospital and the Royal Waterloo Hospital for Women and Children. After a slow start he gradually pursued a career in what became a flourishing and lucrative private practice. His London home, in his latter years as a consultant, 63 Brook Street, had been occupied previously by his former mentor and friend Sir William Jenner. John Williams remained there until he retired in 1903.

In 1886 Queen Victoria, on the recommendation of Sir William, her physician-extraordinary, had invited John Williams to attend the birth of the child of her youngest daughter, Princess Beatrice of Battenberg. It was the beginning of a long and agreeable association with the Royal

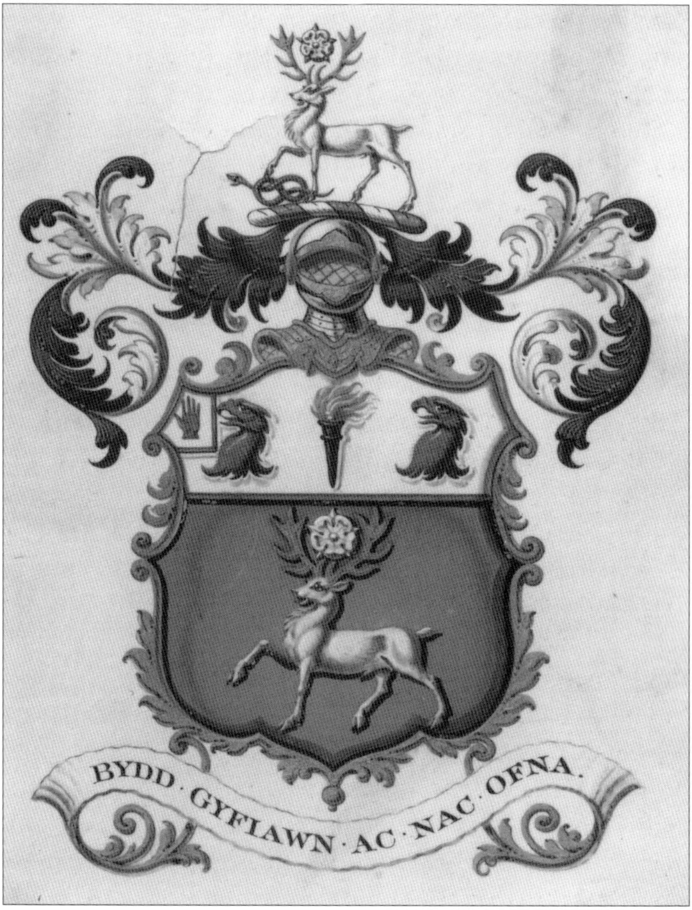

Baronetcy/Coat of Arms.

Family, who held him in high regard: he was to be Physician Accoucheur to the family for many years. In June 1894 he was in attendance when Mary, Duchess of York, gave birth to the future Edward VIII: he was the physician accoucheur for all of Mary's births . . . including that of King George VI.

In October 1894 the Queen granted him a baronetcy: his coat of arms carried the legend 'Bydd gyfiawn, ac nac ofna' ('Be just and fear not').

The Times of 28 March 1895 reported, 'Dinner to Medical Baronets':

> 'A complimentary dinner was given last evening at the Criterion Restaurant to Sir John Erichsen, Sir Russell Reynolds, and Sir John Williams, the recently-created medical baronets.
>
> . . . Sir J. Russell Reynolds said that he stood between his old master, Sir John Erichsen, and his old pupil, Sir John Williams, both of whom he could now happily recognise as old friends . . . Sir John Williams also responded'.

VI

Matters Welsh: Birth of the National Library

The land of his birth was never far from John Williams' mind. He was the chief promoter of a movement to secure funds for the Welsh Hospital Unit sent out to South Africa during the Boer War: Lady Williams had her own 'Collecting Book' for the cause. *The Lancet* of 21 April 1900 records how the Welsh Hospital contingent in the charge of Major Cockerill R.A.M.C. left on 14 April: many friends were at Waterloo Station to see them off, including Sir John, chairman of the committee and Lady Williams. Sir John was also one of the pioneers in the campaign to secure the eradication of tuberculosis in Wales where it was the commonest single cause of death at the beginning of the twentieth century.

But he was also to make very considerable contributions in other areas of Welsh life. In London, he was active in the revived Society of Cymmrodorion: its Record Series gained his support and he was awarded The Cymmrodorion Medal of 1912-1913. He was Vice-President of the Society.

Above all, his early interest in collecting manuscripts, books, prints, art treasures, etc. (particularly those of Welsh interest) informed and encouraged by his friendship with

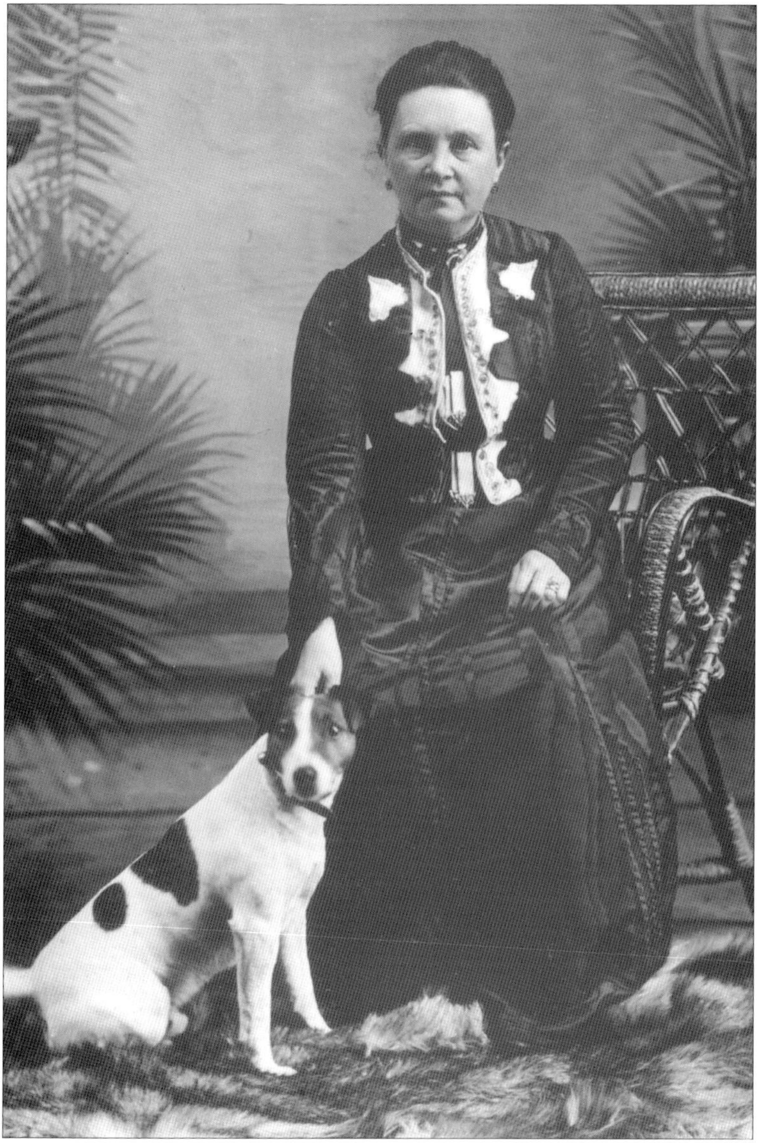

Lady Williams and 'Spot'.

John Deffett Francis, artist and founder of the art gallery and art library at Swansea was to continue throughout his life. He became a discerning collector and sought expert advice – for example from the noted bookseller and publisher Bernard Quaritch of 15 Piccadilly and from Welsh experts such as J. Gwenogvryn Evans, John Humphreys Davies and Henry Owen. The art-dealers and print-sellers in London and many in the provinces were aware of his particular interests. John would either be present himself or be represented at the major book sales. He came to regard his purchases as a foundation collection for a national library in Wales. (But he was more than a 'purchaser': his private papers demonstrate his active interest in matters: for example his notebooks contain a list of books in Welsh or of Welsh matters arranged chronologically, 1546-1894 . . . statistics relating to religious denominations in Wales . . . a transcript of a manuscript containing the poetry of Rhys Prichard . . . histories of the castles of Dinefwr, Dryslwyn, Carreg Cennen, etc. etc. in his own hand.)

The Cymmrodorion Society in the mid-eighteenth century had realised the value of the establishment of a national library for Wales. Richard Morris (1703-1779) founder of the Society had a vision for a national repository and in his will dated 7 November 1773 bequeathed 'to the Governors and Trustees of the British or Welsh School in Gray's Inn Road, my whole valuable collection of ancient British books in print and manuscript, to be deposited in the Library of the said school for the perusal of the curious in British antiquities'. (For reasons of security these were transferred to the British Museum in 1844 and, ultimately, to the British Library.) And from Edward Williams, ('Iolo Morganwg' 1747-1826, stonemason, poet and antiquary)

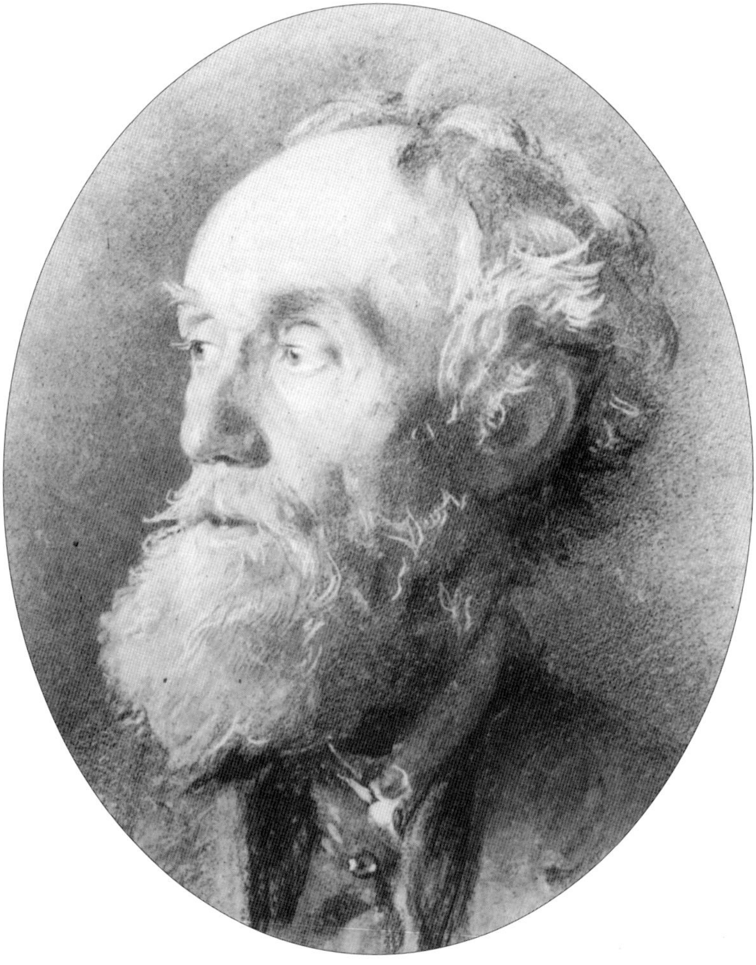

John Deffett Francis.

who travelled far and wide to transcribe and, where possible, to acquire Welsh manuscripts: a 'National Library when founded in Wales (I) will give my MSS to it . . .'. In

1860, Thomas Gee (1815-1898), Calvinistic Methodist minister, journalist and politician, expressed the need for a national library and went as far as to advocate that a petition be presented to Parliament asking for a capital grant of £3,000 to £4,000 to erect a building for the purpose. The idea gained momentum and from the late nineteenth century there was renewed interest in such a possibility. The opening of the University College at Aberystwyth in 1872 provided a focal point. In 1873, a meeting at the National Eisteddfod in Mold had resolved that a national library be established, 'consisting chiefly of rare books and manuscripts in the Welsh language, and in other languages, where they relate to Wales and its people' and the University College was proposed as the first home of such a collection. By 1896 a further Welsh Library Committee was convened there but with the ultimate aim of 'the erection of a library apart from the College for Welsh books, Manuscripts, and Records relating to Wales'.

The outstanding support and tireless campaigning of such prominent Welshmen as Thomas Edward Ellis, John Herbert Lewis, Daniel Lleufer Thomas, John Humphreys Davies, Alfred Thomas and Henry Owen together with the ultimate commitment which Lloyd George was to give to ensure that the Library should have parity with similar institutions in the United Kingdom were fundamental to its existence. Parliament, Cymmrodorion, Eisteddfod were to be vital platforms for pleading and the fact that a nucleus Welsh library existed at the University College in Aberystwyth, served with devotion by its librarian J. Glyn Davies, all advanced the cause. The foundation of the Chair of Celtic at the University of Oxford in 1877, the passing of the Welsh Intermediate School Act in 1889, the creation of a 'University of Wales' comprising colleges at Aberystwyth, Bangor and Cardiff in 1893, the Central Welsh Board in 1895 and the Welsh Department of Education in 1907 all pointed in a particular direction. Leading Welshmen exuded confidence in the prospect of national institutions: they shared something of the climate of optimism and progressiveness of the time and in a renewed awareness of Welsh national identity.

But, the endeavours of Sir John Williams – his personal contacts, his public pronouncements and appearances and, above all, his willingness to contribute his vast treasure of collected items – were to prove decisive, not only in establishing the national library but also in securing its being located at Aberystwyth (a location supported by Lloyd George).

Such endeavours, together with those of his coterie of co-workers, counteracted the claims of other locations, Cardiff in particular. After much public debate the Privy Council announced on 10 June 1905 that a National Museum be established in Cardiff and a National Library in Aberystwyth. (Characteristically Sir John penned a telegram of congratulation to the Mayor and Corporation of Cardiff on securing the National Museum there.) On 19 March 1907 each was granted a royal charter. The infant Library's temporary home from January 1909 was the 1820s Assembly Rooms in Laura Place, with John Ballinger as Librarian.

Ballinger, forty-eight-year-old, was the energetic, far-sighted, well-established and successful librarian of the Cardiff Free Library. There is no doubt that he would have liked to have seen the National Library situated at Cardiff, recognising the advantage of the splendid collection there including material from the E. R. G. Salisbury and Sir Thomas Phillipps libraries. Ballinger may well have acquiesced as a result of his great respect for and admiration of Sir John Williams: maybe he had been secretly promised the post at Aberystwyth. He was appointed there at a salary of £600 per annum. It was a brilliant coup.

Ahead was the arduous work of securing capital and annual grants. John Williams chaired the Appeal Fund, directed operations and continued to engage the cooperation of devoted fellow-Welshmen – none more so than Daniel Lleufer Thomas who proved to be an outstanding money-raiser.

Sir John was to preside at the laying of the foundation stone of the Library on 15 July 1911 by King George V and Queen Mary on the incomparable, elevated site overlooking the town of Aberystwyth. (The site on Grogythan Hill purchased by Lord Rendel in 1897 was donated by him as the site for the National Library. Stuart Rendel, industrialist, politician, philanthropist was an Englishman, educated at Eton and Oriel College, Oxford, who had entered Parliament in 1880 and soon became Leader of the Welsh members there and a prime promoter of matters of Welsh interest.) The King bestowed on Sir John the Grand Cross of the Victorian Order in appreciation of his work on behalf of the Library. (King Edward VII had honoured him with the K.C.V.O. in 1902 and the King of Denmark had conferred on him the Grand Cross of the Order of Dannebrog in 1903.) The King also conferred the Order of St Andrew on John Ballinger, the Librarian.

In that year, 1911, the Library was granted the status of a Deposit Library under the Copyright Act. It was a vital step in the growth of the new institution giving it entitlement of

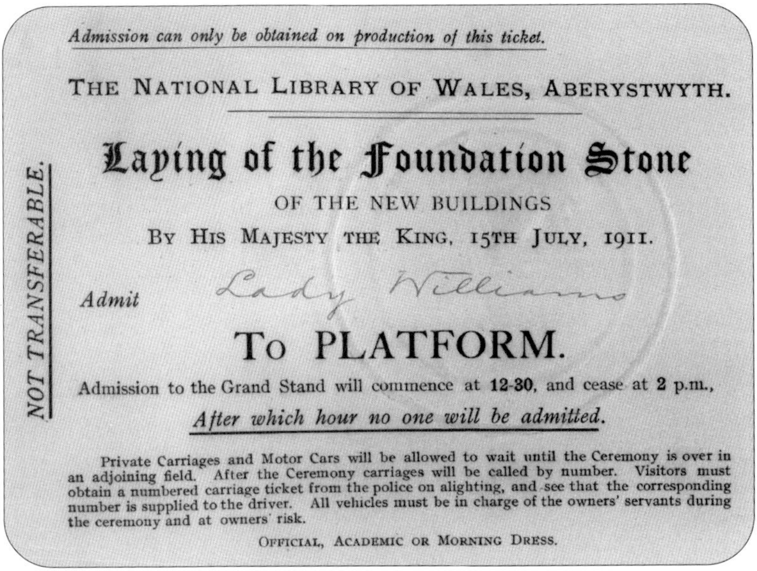

Admission can only be obtained on production of this ticket.

NOT TRANSFERABLE.

THE NATIONAL LIBRARY OF WALES, ABERYSTWYTH.

Laying of the Foundation Stone

OF THE NEW BUILDINGS

BY HIS MAJESTY THE KING, 15TH JULY, 1911.

Admit Lady Williams

To PLATFORM.

Admission to the Grand Stand will commence at **12-30**, and cease at **2** p.m.,

After which hour no one will be admitted.

Private Carriages and Motor Cars will be allowed to wait until the Ceremony is over in an adjoining field. After the Ceremony carriages will be called by number. Visitors must obtain a numbered carriage ticket from the police on alighting, and see that the corresponding number is supplied to the driver. All vehicles must be in charge of the owners' servants during the ceremony and at owners' risk.

OFFICIAL, ACADEMIC OR MORNING DRESS.

The Ceremony: Laying the Foundation Stone.

one copy of all books, magazines, maps and other printed material produced in the United Kingdom and Ireland. Securing this owed so much to the diplomacy of the Vice-President, John Herbert Lewis, M.P. for Flint Boroughs . . . and to the persistence of John Ballinger. And it was John Herbert Lewis – who had served the cause of the Library with such dogged determination over the years – with John Humphreys Davies who accompanied Sir John in a deputation to the Chancellor of the Exchequer, David Lloyd George, seeking financial support towards the new building on Grogythan Hill.

It was four years later that parts of the new building were sufficiently ready for taking the books: they were transferred by horse and wagon between August 1915 and St David's

Day 1916.

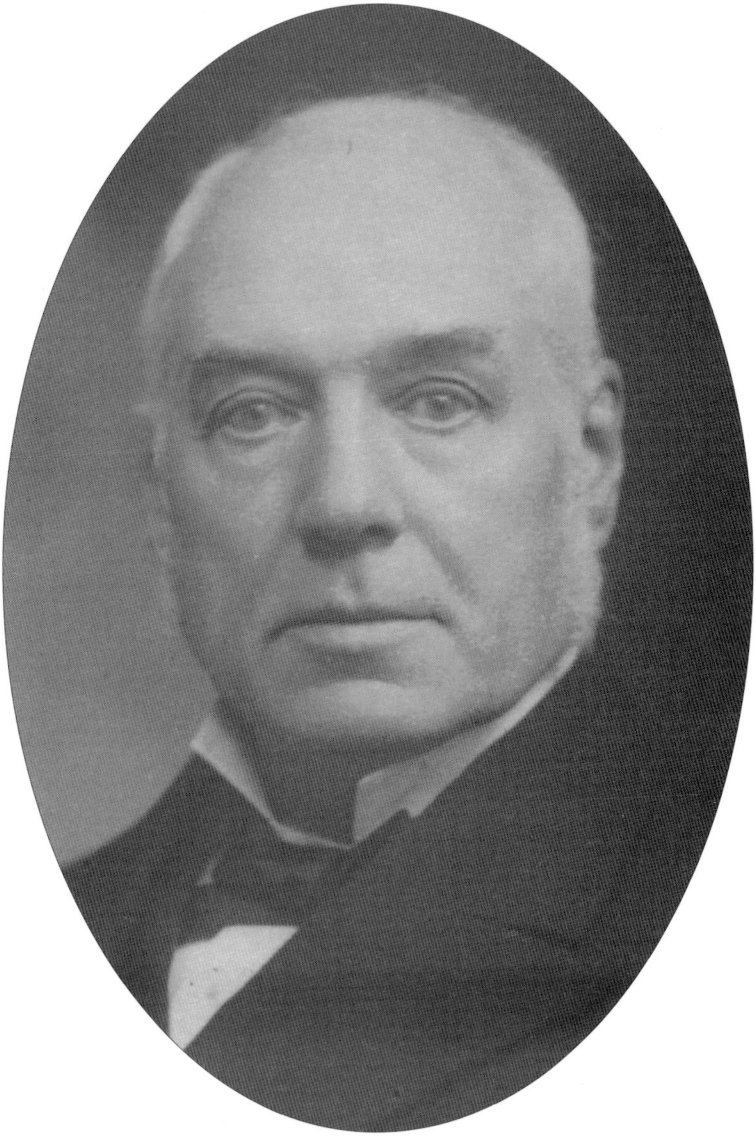

Sir John Williams, Bart.

VII

Bequests

It was entirely appropriate, when the Library received its Charter in 1907, that Sir John Williams, its principal founder and benefactor, should have been nominated as its first President. The collection of some 1,200 manuscripts, 25,000 books and the many prints, drawings, etc. which he presented was priceless, including as it did vital manuscript collections of early Welsh poetry and prose, together with invaluable manuscript material of later centuries. The earliest printed books were there, together with a host of later publications. Apart from the judicious individual collecting over the years, aided by the advice of friends and mentors, Sir John was able to acquire really major collections: for example the Shirburn Castle collection of books (and manuscripts) sold to him, 1898-1900 and the Hengwrt-Peniarth collection, purchased in 1904 (*the* collection that tipped the balance in favour of Aberystwyth as the location for the National Library). Such acquisitions not only made Sir John the premier Welsh book-collector but it also demonstrated the urgency of having a library to house such a collection.

The Shirburn Castle collection, which had been seen by the expert palaeographer J. Gwenogvryn Evans and by John Humphreys Davies in 1898 was a library assembled by the Reverend Samuel Williams (*c.*1660-*c.*1722) who had acquired a talent as a copyist of manuscripts, and more particularly his son, the Reverend Moses Williams, F.R.S. (1685-1742) who had been an assistant to Edward Lhuyd at the Ashmolean Museum in Oxford and later served on the staff of the Bodleian Library there. Moses Williams had visited the great houses of Wales, examining their libraries and copying from their manuscripts.

The Hengwrt-Peniarth collection had originally been assembled by that remarkable antiquary and collector, Robert Vaughan of Hengwrt (*c.*1592-1667). It passed to William Watkin Edward Wynne (1801-1880) of Peniarth, near Tywyn, Merioneth in 1859, a Member of Parliament but best remembered as an antiquary, genealogist and custodian of the Hengwrt collection. The collection had been examined and catalogued by J. Gwenogvryn Evans who described it as 'undoubtedly the premier collection of Welsh manuscripts both in extent and quality'. The *South Wales Daily News* of 4 May 1904 reported 'well founded rumours that Sir John had become purchaser of the Peniarth Library. If true, Aberystwyth has already been placed absolutely beyond competition, in regard to the promised Welsh National Library . . .'. The Hengwrt-Peniarth collection was ultimately to become Sir John's, and the Library's, in February 1909.

There were other interesting purchases, for example, in 1894 Sir John had acquired some sixty manuscripts from the scholar Egerton Phillimore (1856-1937). (Phillimore was to keep close contact with him: the numerous references in Sir John's papers to Phillimore's finances and acknowledgement of receipt of cheques confirm this.) In 1895 Sir John purchased one hundred and forty items from the Middle Hill collection of Sir Thomas Phillipps (1792-1872) of Broadway, Worcestershire, the largest private collector of his day. (One manuscript of the Phillipps' collection which did not come into Sir John's possession was *The Book of Aneirin,* a vital manuscript containing a heroic poem accredited to the poet Aneirin who flourished in the latter part of the sixth century. This 'book' was purchased by the Cardiff Free Libraries Committee in 1896.)

Sir John also bought the library of John Parry (1835-1897) of Llanarmon-yn-Iâl, a man of scant education but a book-collector and a voracious reader particularly in the field of Puritan theology, political and church history: it was primarily a Welsh language collection comprising 4,558 volumes including periodicals.

The consequence, particularly as a result of the Hengwrt-Peniarth and Shirburn Castle purchases, was an archive of immense importance which Sir John Williams was to bequeath. It included *Historia Regum Britanniae* ('The History of the Kings of Britain') *c.*1136 by Geoffrey of Monmouth, *The Black Book of Carmarthen, c.*1250+, containing the oldest manuscript collection of Welsh poetry, *The Black Book of Chirk,* dating from the mid-thirteenth century, containing one of the earliest Welsh language versions of the Laws of Hywel Dda, *The Book of Taliesin,* early fourteenth century, including poems ascribed to Taliesin who flourished in the late sixth century, *The White Book of Rhydderch,* mid-fourteenth century, containing a collection of Welsh prose including texts of the Mabinogion tales and *The Red Book of Talgarth* written *c.*1400 by Hywel Fychan ap Howel Goch of Builth. Among the bequest too were the earliest Welsh printed books: *Yny Lhyvyr Hwnn* (1546), a manual of instruction in the principles of the Christian faith by Sir

John Price, *Oll Synnwyr Pen* (1547) a collection of proverbs compiled by William Salesbury, *A Dictionary in Englyshe and Welshe* (1547) by Salesbury, *Testament Newydd* (1567) mainly by Salesbury and the first Welsh *Bible* (1588) by William Morgan. Among many other treasures was the rare Welsh grammar of Gruffydd Robert, printed at Milan in 1567.

There were, too, almanacs, ballads, tracts and a host of graphic works of Welsh relevance – maps, plans, prints, drawings and portraits. (In 1898, for example, Sir John had purchased a set of prints and drawings of Wales by S. H. Grimm and eighty-four plates of Buck's views of Wales . . . in 1908 a set of forty-eight topographical drawings made in 1796 during Thomas Rowlandson's tour in Wales.)

In addition, there were other treasures – some rare Cornish manuscripts (among them the unique text of a mystery play relating the *Life of St Meriasek*, written in 1504), a number of French manuscripts dating from the fourteenth to the nineteenth century (including four early Arthurian tales in French) and an illuminated Passional of the late fifteenth century *La Passion de nostre saulueur Jhesucrist* in thirty-six chapters. There were English gems such as a twelfth century text of Bede's *Ecclesiastica Historia Gentes Anglorum*, one of the two earliest manuscript texts of Geoffrey Chaucer's *Canterbury Tales*, early editions of Thomas Malory and the English Holinshed *Chronicles* of 1577. Because of Sir John's interest in fine printing he had collected most of the Kelmscott Press publications (the press established by William Morris whose designs featured in so many items of furniture in Sir John and Lady Williams' home in Aberystwyth).

Here have been noted only a sample of Sir John's bequests. They would have exceeded, by far, the dreams of those who had proposed a national library for Wales at the National Eisteddfod of 1873.

* * *

After Sir John's death many of the pictures which hung on the walls of his Aberystwyth home, together with engravings, photographs, water-colours and oil-paintings passed to the Library. The house, on the promenade, and much of the furnishings were left to the University College.

VIII

Llanstephan . . . Aberystwyth

By 1904 Sir John had returned to Wales from London: Lady Williams and he resided at the Plas, Llanstephan, in Carmarthenshire, overlooking the Tywi estuary. He became involved in county affairs – as Justice of the Peace, as High Sheriff (appointed in 1904), as founding member of the

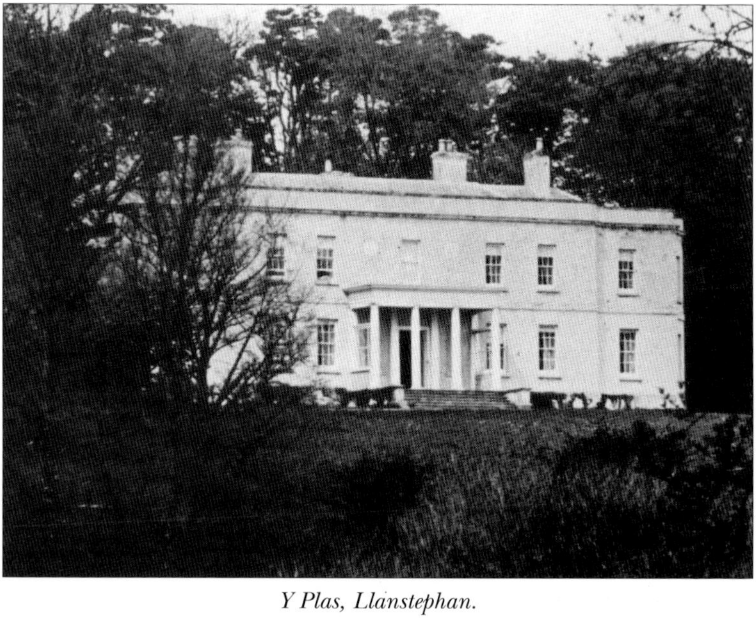

Y Plas, Llanstephan.

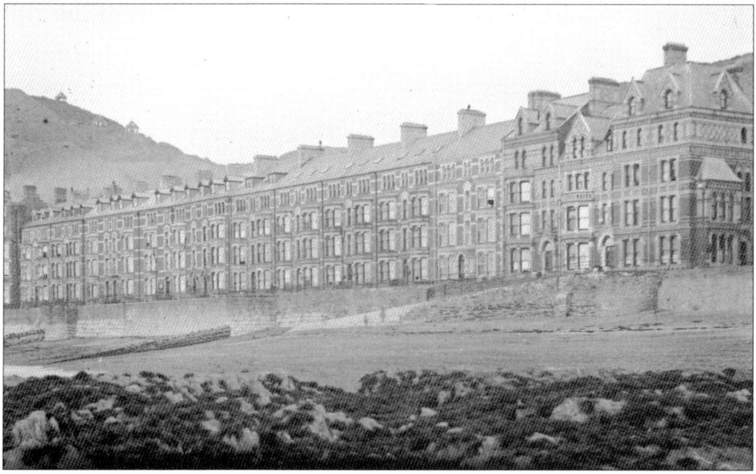

Victoria Terrace, Aberystwyth.

Carmarthenshire Antiquarian Society in 1905. In May 1906 he was appointed a member of the Royal Commission on the Disestablishment of the Church in Wales.

In November 1908 John Ballinger had visited Llanstephan to discuss with Sir John the removal of the collection of 24,500 volumes weighing some twelve tons, to the Assembly Rooms in Aberystwyth. The removal took place in January 1909.

The location for the National Library housing his remarkable collection enticed him to Aberystwyth. He and Lady Williams moved to 'Snowdon Villa', Victoria Terrace, on the sea-front, in September 1909: he re-named the house *Blaenllynant,* in memory of his childhood home. (It was John Humphreys Davies the registrar of the college who had found the house for them.) In 1910, he was appointed Honorary Colonel in the Royal Army Medical Corps, Welsh Territorial Division.

Clearly, no appointment pleased him more than his presidency of the National Library: when he intimated in 1911 that it was time to relinquish his post, the Vice-President, Sir John Herbert Lewis reminded him, '. . . you are the Father of the Library and as long as you live you must remain the head of the family'.

Sir John had continued over the years to collect and to use his very considerable organising talents, tact, contacts, energy – and what Daniel Huws former keeper of the Manuscripts called 'his powers of persuasion' – towards the well-being of the Library. He was described as being of average height, of robust build, quiet, friendly, entertaining, possessing the perfect 'bedside manner': he was fond of country life, enjoying such pursuits as fishing and shooting.

He and Lady Williams were remembered as being excellent hosts. Dr David Jenkins who joined the staff of the Library in 1939 and served as Librarian from 1969 until 1979 was to refer to him as 'a singularly great man'.

Lord Rendel died in June 1913 and Sir John, who had been Honorary Treasurer from 1899 to 1906 and Vice-President from 1906 to 1913 succeeded him as President of the University College at Aberystwyth, a position – together with that of the Library – which he held until his death. (He chaired the meeting of the College Council in 1920 which elected his 'adviser' and friend John Humphreys Davies to the principalship.) With his life-long interest in education, scientific education in particular, and his readiness to promote the study of the language, literature and history of Wales, he was able to use his talents and experience to good effect in serving the university.

Lady Williams predeceased him in 1915: there were no children of the marriage. In 1919 Thomas David Jenkins commissioned the Italian sculptor, Professor Mario Rutelli, to sculpt a marble statue of Sir John: it was carved from a single block of Carrara marble, presented to the Library Court on 3 October 1924 and unveiled by Lady Herbert Lewis. For some years Sir John's health had been failing. His last public duty at the Library was to open the very first exhibition to be held in the new exhibition gallery – now the Gregynog Gallery – on 5 June 1920: appropriately it was an exhibition of manuscripts and printed books which Sir John had acquired. The Court of Governors presented him with an illuminated address to mark his eightieth birthday on 6 November 1920 and to acknowledge his great service to the Library.

Sir John Williams died on 24 May 1926 and was buried at Aberystwyth on 27 May at a private funeral, the service being led by the Reverend Dr Peter Price, pastor of Baker Street Welsh Congregational Chapel of which Sir John was a member. The Librarian, John Ballinger, was among the mourners. A memorial service was held some days later with addresses by Professor Edward Edwards, Vice-Principal of the University College and Sir Evan Davies Jones, Treasurer of the National Library (and soon to be its Vice-President). The King and Queen had sent a message of sympathy expressing sorrow at 'the death of their old and trusted friend'.

In his will Sir John bequeathed very substantial sums of money to both the Library and the University. The university utilised part of the money to promote Welsh studies. The 'Sir John Williams Chair of Welsh History' was created in 1930 to honour his memory. There was a particular appropriateness to this in that it was he who had offered to pay the cost of a research lectureship in Welsh History in 1910. And in all probability it was Sir John who had financed a Readership in Welsh Literature in 1912: T. Gwynn Jones was appointed its first incumbent in 1913. The Library used its bequest towards the completion of the Administrative Block and other projects: Sir John had already made very substantial contributions to the Building Fund.

*   *   *

Sir John Williams had been awarded honorary doctorates by the universities of Glasgow, Aberdeen, Edinburgh and Wales. He was, and is, revered not only as a distinguished physician of his day but as one of the all-time outstanding benefactors of Wales. Dr J. Gwenogvryn Evans dedicated his facsimile of *The Black Book of Carmarthen*, 1907, in this way: 'The First President of the Welsh National Library, the first in personal effort for its establishment, the first in personal sacrifice for its good, and the first in the importance of his contribution to its treasures'. Margot, Countess of Oxford, who had been his patient, commented, 'Sir John . . . would have been a remarkable man in any country, but in Wales he stands alone'. Princess Maud, grand-daughter of Queen Victoria (later Queen Maud of Norway, consort of King Haakon), addressed him in these words, 'We shall never forget your great kindness to us. Believe me'. The people of Wales could hardly put it better: the National Library remains his perennial monument.

Appendices

APPENDIX A

The Williams Family

There were five children:

1. DAVID (1833-1862). Remained at home to farm Blaenllynant. He helped to build CAPEL MAEN, the daughter church of JERUSALEM which with its 369 members in 1851 was too small to accommodate, and not convenient for the wide area. CAPEL MAEN was opened in 1853: David was its first secretary. He was buried at Bethlehem Chapel.
2. MORGAN (1835-1918). He emigrated to the USA, fought in the Civil War and died in Harford, Maryland, in 1918 without issue. His estate passed to the one surviving brother, Sir John Williams.
3. MARY ELISABETH (1837-1841). Died suddenly and buried at Bethlehem Chapel.
4. JOHN (1840-1926).
5. NATHANIEL (1843-1908). Like John, attended the Normal School, Swansea. He worked on the farm at Blaenllynant and with David helped to support CAPEL MAEN: he also became its secretary. His mother assigned Blaenllynant to him on a 21 year lease at £90 per annum in 1873. Later he and his wife Elizabeth moved to Glandules, Llangathen, Llandeilo. He died without issue in 1908 and his estate, too, passed to Sir John Williams.

APPENDIX B

The Eleanor Williams Exhibition

'It is very gratifying to find a true revival of the good old-fashioned personal interest in education, manifested in the form of grants to aid deserving but poor scholars. We have now the pleasure to report that Dr John Williams, of London, the eminent obstetrician – who was for some years resident in Swansea, and who married the daughter of Richard Hughes, Esq., J.P., Ynistawe, – has decided to benefit his native county by founding an educational exhibition. Dr John Williams proposes to establish an exhibition to be called the Eleanor Williams Exhibition, to be competed for by boys from any Elementary School within the Parishes of Llangadock, Llanddeusant, Myddfau, Llansadwrn, and Llanwrda, in the County of Carmarthen. The object of the exhibition is to enable deserving lads to proceed to, and continue their education at, a Higher-grade School, such as the Welsh Collegiate Institution, Llandovery, or Christ's College, Brecon. The exhibition will be of the annual value of £25, and tenable for four years, provided the holder produces at the end of each school term a certificate from his head master of satisfactory progress and good conduct. The first competition will take place at Llangadock, in September 1885. Intending candidates must not be more than 14 years of age on September 1, 1885. In cases of equality, preference will be given to a native of Llangadock.

The subjects of the examination will be arithmetic, English, reading, grammar and analysis, history and poetry, Euclid book 1, algebra, Welsh reading and translation from Welsh to English. – It will be remembered that it was Dr Williams who was the means of presenting to the Swansea Public Library the celebrated print of Hogarth recently. It is all very well to ask and wait for Government aid towards education, but private self sacrificing effort is far more potent if those who are able to do so would follow the example so well set by Dr Williams of London.'

From *The Cambrian*, Swansea, March 13, 1885)

APPENDIX C

Publications

1. Transactions of The Obstetric Society:

1876 'Mechanical action of pessaries'.

1877 'Pathology and treatment of membranous dysmenorrhoea'.

1882 Monograph on natural history of dysmenorrhoea.

1884 'On the circulation in the uterus, with some of its anatomical and pathological bearings'.

1884 'Note on corroding ulcer of os uteri, with an account of the post-mortem findings'.

1885 'Notes on serous perimetritis'.

1887 Presidential year, 'during which he distinguished himself greatly, by the skilful content of discussions, and foresaw how ephemeral would be the fame of Apostoli's method, then attracting great interest'. This year also, he delivered the Harveian oration, and spoke on 'Cancer of Uterus'.

1897 Cavendish lectures on 'Ovarian tumours complicating pregnancy'.

Reynolds *System of Medicine* had articles on growths of uterus, tumours of ovary, and ovarian inflamations, contributed by John Williams.

(Taken from 'The Medical Aspect of the Life of Sir John Williams, Bart., G.C.V.O., M.D., F.R.C.P., 1840-1926', by Iorwerth Hughes Jones, *National Library of Wales Journal*, 1955-56).

The Lancet
(various contributions by John Williams):

1873 'The physical changes in the position of the healthy unimpregnated uterus'.

1873-1880 'On the mechanism of production of certain displacements of the uterus'.

1878 'Ovariotomy performed on the antiseptic method the patient being in a state of pyrexia: recovery'.

1881 A letter (written from Harley Street) concerning 'Dr Braxton-Hicks on intermittent contractions of the uterus'.

1890 The opening address in Obstetrics at the International Medical Congress at Berlin on 'The total extirpation of the uterus by the vagina'.

APPENDIX D

Funeral at Aberystwyth

The funeral of Sir John Williams, Bart., G.C.V.O., took place at Aberystwyth on Thursday week, and was of a private nature. Interment was made at Aberystwyth Cemetery and the Rev. Peter Price, D.D., pastor of Baker Street Welsh Congregational Church, of which Sir John was a member, officiated at the house and graveside.

The mourners were Miss Annie Lewis, Miss S. Lewis, North-road, cousins: Mrs Williams, Beili Gwynfe, Llandovery, cousin; and Mr David Williams J.P., Beili Gwynfe; Mr David Williams, Dryslwyn, cousin; Mr J. W. Nicholas, clerk to Carmarthenshire County Council, cousin, and Mrs Nicholas; Mr R. E. Jones, Oakely Grange, Shrewsbury, cousin; Mr Edward Hughes, Mathafarn, Cemmaes, cousin; Mr and Mrs J. P. Owen, Blaenllynant, Mrs Peter Price, Mrs Timothy Lewis; Mr John Ballinger, C.B.E., M.A., Librarian of the National Library: Mr David Ellis; Mr Evan Evans, Solicitor, and Mr J. W. P. Parry, Aberystwyth.

Mrs Hughes, Sir John's mother-in-law, and Principal J. H. Davies were present at the house but owing to ill-health were unable to attend the funeral.

The coffin bore the inscription "Sir John Williams, Bart. Died May 24th, 1926, aged 86 years".

*　　*　　*

Royal Sympathy

Principal J. H. Davies, M.A., of the University College of Wales, has received a letter from the private secretary to Queen Mary, stating how sorry were both Their Majesties the King and Queen to hear of the death of their old and trusted friend, Sir John Williams

(From *The Cambrian News*, June 4, 1926)

APPENDIX E

Tributes

SIR JOHN WILLIAMS

Tribute to a Great Man

ABERYSTWYTH MEMORIAL SERVICE

Tributes to the memory of Sir John Williams, Bart., G.C.V.O., LL.D., M.D., D.Sc., president of the National Library of Wales and of the University College of Wales, Aberystwyth, were paid at a memorial service at the University Hall, Aberystwyth, on Sunday.

The service was attended by the Mayor, Corporation and officials, and the staff of the College in academic dress. Among those on the platform were the Rev. Dr Peter Price, Canon Williams, Sir Evan D. Jones, treasurer of the National Library, Sir Francis Edwards, Mr John Ballinger, C.B.E., librarian of the National Library . . . Mr G. Eyre Evans . . .

The service was conducted by the Rev. Peter Price, D.D., and the Rev. Canon David Williams, M.A. The singing was led by the UCW small choir and accompanied by a small orchestra, Dr D. de Lloyd being the conductor, Mr Chas H. Clements, Mus. Bac. F.R.C.O., was the accompanist.

When the small choir had sung the 23rd Psalm the large congregation sang "*Ar lan Iorddonen ddofn . . .*"

Vice-Principal Edward Edwards, M.A., then gave the following Welsh address:

"Nid Marw"

. . . Llywydd ein Coleg, dinesydd enwocaf ein tref, y gŵr a gerid gan bawb, i'r hwn nad oedd un gelyn yn unman – y mae tristwch am dano yng nghalon Cymru gyfan a wyneb ein cenedl yn wlyb gan ei dagrau. Canys yr oedd Syr John yn ddyn rhy fawr i fyw o fewn terfyn na phlaid, na sect – ei wlad, ei Gymru, ei hangen a'i gobaith, ei haddysg, a'i chrefydd oedd testun cyson ei feddwl a'i ofal ar hyd ei oes.

. . . yr oedd ei ysbryd yn isel a syml, y dyn hawddaf i fyned ato . . . Treuliodd ran helaeth o'i fywyd yng ngwlad estron, ond yr oedd ei heniaith ei hun yn lân ar ei wefus . . . a'i barch i'w fam a'i magodd . . . yn rhamant sanctaidd yn ei hanes. Yr oedd yn foneddwr wrth natur, hardd ei berson, hardd ei ysbryd . . . Cafodd fyw yn hir, drwy drugaredd fawr, bywyd o aberth difwlch a chymwynas ddidor i'w wlad, bywyd o gasglu trysorau yr hen oesoedd er mwyn cyfoethogi meddwl yr oes hon.

* * *

Sir Evan Jones said:

. . . this vast audience which speaks volumes . . . What I want to say . . . is something with regard to the personal greatness of Sir John Williams as exemplified by that great institution of which he is the father and which you in Aberystwyth have the honour of having placed among you. I do not wish to speak of the National Library as the cause of, or, even the partial cause of the greatness of the man. I rather wish to speak of it as a product of his greatness. This great institution owes its being to the man we are here tonight to commemorate. He nursed it during its infancy; he supported it from the years of adolescence, and he brought it to the splendid position which it occupies today.

. . . He was a great humanist and he was a great Welsh patron . . . He had great constancy of purpose and he had a great and deep love for his native land. These characteristics found expression in the National Library which he brought into life.

. . . He was collecting great treasures, not for his own gratification not only as a lad or for amusement and enjoyment, but as part of his scheme for benefiting his fellow men and especially his fellow countrymen.

. . . The place of a great library in the life of a nation was to him a supreme thought, a supreme guidance, something which he used as an object to be aimed at; and his object was to bring within the reach of Welshmen those facilities for higher studies which he believed to be one of the fundamental needs of Wales. How splendidly he succeeded. It was to him a great and constant happiness that he lived to see realised his great idea of a centre of intellectual life and its future assured. . . . He created enthusiasm in others . . .

(Sir Evan was there in place of Sir John Herbert Lewis who had suffered an accident).

A letter from JH-L:

> The noble building which towers above Aberystwyth will stand for centuries as a monument to the founder of the National Library . . . it was an honour and a privilege to serve under such a chief.

Sir Evan D. Jones:

> . . . a man of tenacious purpose, gifted far above the average, tactful, gracious, kind and generous, dominated throughout his life by a desire to serve the highest interests of his country. He loved Wales and everything Welsh.
>
> . . . He has earned and will ever retain a predominant place amongst the great men of his own country . . . He has bequeathed to his countrymen a kingdom in the realm of culture of no mean dimensions.

(Excerpts from *The Cambrian News* and *Farmers Gazette*, June 4, 1926)

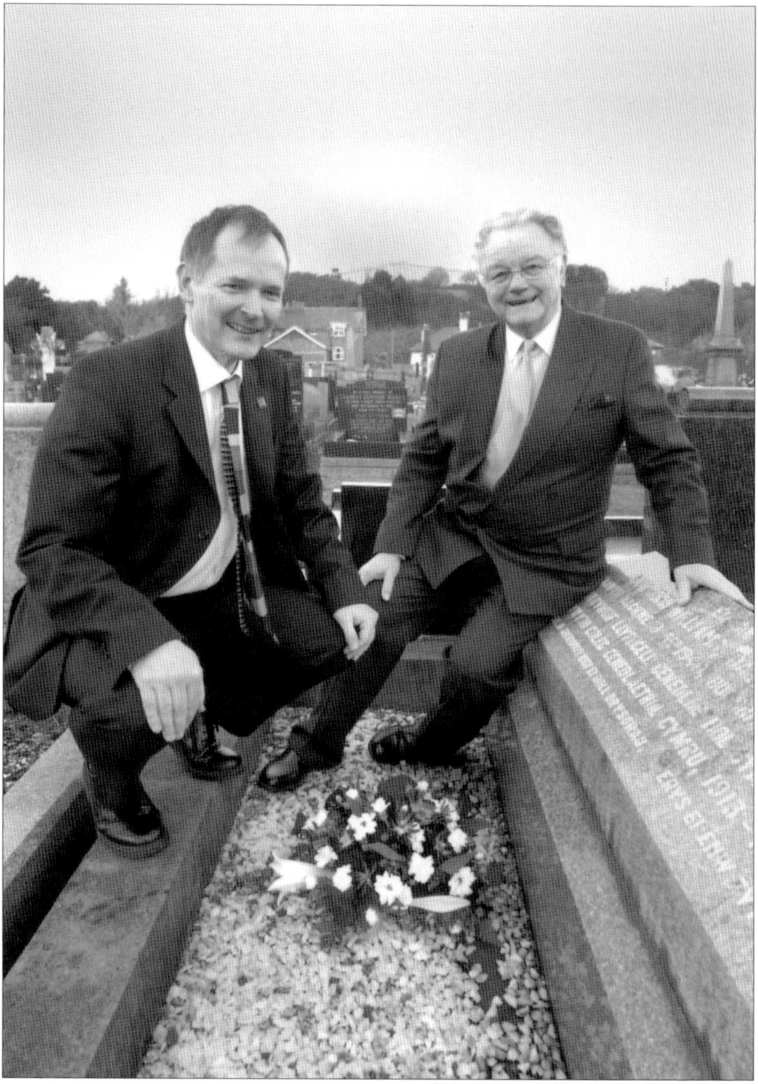

The President and the Librarian laying a wreath on the grave of Sir John and Lady Williams on 19 March 2007, the centenary of the granting of the Royal Charter.

APPENDIX F

The Gravestone of Sir John and Lady Williams at Aberystwyth Cemetery

Er cof am
Yr Arglwyddes Mary Elizabeth Anne Williams
Gwraig Syr John Williams, Barwnig M.D.,
Ganwyd Chwefror 7fed 1850
bu farw Mawrth 1af 1915

Er cof am
Syr John Williams, Barwnig, G.C.V.O.
Ganwyd Tachwedd 6ed 1840, hunodd Mai 24ain 1926
Llywydd cyntaf Llyfrgell Genedlaethol Cymru
1907-1926
Llywydd Coleg Cenedlaethol Cymru
1913-1926

Carodd ei genedl a rhoddodd iddi ei holl drysorau.
Erys ei enw fyth yn annwyl.

APPENDIX G

Select Bibliography

The National Library of Wales Journal, Vol. 1, No. 4. (1940).

Ruth Evans, *John Williams 1840-1926* (1952).

David Jenkins, *A Refuge in Peace and War: The National Library of Wales to 1952* (2002).

W. LL. D(avies), *Sir John Williams (1840-1926) Dictionary of Welsh Biography* (1959).

W. LL. Davies, *The National Library of Wales* (1937).

Emyr Wyn Jones, 'Sir John Williams (1840-1926) His Background and Achievement', in John Cule (ed.) *Wales and Medicine* (1975).

R. Brinley Jones, *The National Library of Wales 1907-2007,* Cambria Volume 9, Number 2, June–July 2007.

E. L. Ellis, *The University College of Wales, Aberystwyth 1872-1972* (1972).

Kenneth O. Morgan, *Wales in British Politics 1868-1922* (1980).

Sir John Williams: Deeds and Papers, National Library of Wales.